Harper

Harper

48 Days to Change the Lives of Millions

By William Stanfield

BELLE ISLE BOOKS

ISBN: 978-1-9399302-0-0

Library of Congress Control Number: 2014936018

Printed in the United States

Published by

BELLE ISLE BOOKS

www.belleislebooks.com

To the doctors, nurses, family, friends, Facebookers, and community, but most of all to Harper, our TooT, without whom Mommy and I would not know just how strong a parent's love for a child can be.

Saying Hello

I n the twenty-fourth week of our first and only pregnancy, my girlfriend, Erin, and I discovered that our unborn daughter had a serious physical defect called a congenital diaphragmatic hernia (or CDH). After consulting with specialists, we learned that this meant a hole in her diaphragm was allowing organs from her abdomen to move into her chest cavity. In other words, we were about to start a long, painful struggle full of surgeries and treatments to keep our daughter, Harper, alive.

The words "it's hard" sound so trivial in such a time of suspense and mortal danger. No one can prepare you for the emotional distress, physical exhaustion, or the sheer volume of facts and knowledge you have to digest when it comes to witnessing your child in such a vulnerable state. The time, money, and resources you have to juggle come second to the well-being of your counterpart, family, and most of all, your child.

There are many kinds of parental pain I don't know. I won't pretend to know what it's like to see your child disappointed, ridiculed, or rejected. I don't know what it's like to see your child's heart broken by the "love of their life." Unfortunately, I can regurgitate how it feels to see tubes, wiring, and machinery working simultaneously to save my daughter's life.

Tears of despair, happiness, and hope all seem to feel the same. Smiles, frowns, blank stares, and faces of confusion blend together like watercolors on a canvas. Emotions become meaningless blurs, like the faces in car windows as they speed by. It is not about you anymore. Days of not knowing how to react to your girlfriend being pregnant are over. You are at home plate, now step up.

These words could be no truer, but at the same time how the hell do you just go into something like this? You don't. No one can tell you what to expect—it just happens. Minute by minute, your world changes, and hour by hour, you're hoping for the best but expecting the worst. It's much like a chess game . . . one wrong move and your world will crumble, and the kingdom you defend will fall.

As time wore on, day-to-day activities that we had always taken for granted began to slip away, and I found myself constantly asking, "What did I do today?" Something as simple as grocery shopping would morph itself into a complicated mess of finding out what would and would not be a waste of money. Trivial as that may seem, the stresses of such minor details mounted upon themselves, waiting to erupt like a volcano. Bickering became the norm at the same time that fights became nonexistent, not because we had nothing to argue about, but because exhaustion held us back.

Eventually all of that stress would force its escape, and we would break down and cry. Fortunately, this release provided a small measure of salvation: the ability to smile, and the renewed strength to start the cycle over again.

As a father, the stress of not being able to defend my child from danger drove me insane. I tried constantly to find answers that did not exist and ways to protect her that did not work. The only thing I could do was attempt the daunting task of patience.

Truth be told, I'm impatient with very few things. I try to look for the good within the bad. But constant reminders that your child is in pain and fighting for her life wear on you. The more I learned of the trials facing her, the more I experienced a harsh numbness overtaking me—not for a lack of caring, but out of necessity. You begin to feel like you are morphing into this thoughtless parent, but you have to remind yourself that you are only looking for the good in all of this.

And then there was my feeling of helplessness in the face of her mother's pain. Nights went by when her mother cried and uttered the words, "I don't feel like a parent." What the hell do you say to that? Nothing. You don't offer kind words of "It will be okay," because you never know that it will be. The only thing to do is hold her and let the concern drain from her body one tear at a time.

I have often wondered if just the sight of me reminds her of Harper, and whether that is a good or bad thing, and for sanity's sake, I pray it is for the better. Testimonies of child traumas tearing parents apart can't help but resonate in the back of my mind, and I often have to remind myself that all of this is real.

News of Erin's pregnancy shocked many, including myself. Suspicions of pregnancy rattled in my brain for months—yes, months—before we both received confirmation. I blame fear as the cause for delayed testing, but after hints became discussions and nudges became pushes, an obstetrician visit was imminent. The words "you're pregnant" were met with smiles, nerves, and an overwhelming feeling of awe. It would be weeks before we learned the darker side of this news.

My own childhood was nothing to write home about. It was filled with obstacles, sadness, and despair; however, if anyone asked me whether I would change it, without batting an eye, I would say no. As a family, we charged through hell and back again, and I promised myself early on that I would be a loving father. Of course, I never knew that fatherhood would prove so challenging from the very start. Still, becoming a father was, and will forever be, the most magical experience of my life.

Luckily for Erin, her pregnancy was relatively painless. Morning sickness and all the other troubling effects didn't come into play. Of course, she would have gladly accepted puking, swollen ankles, and the occasional hemorrhoid if it meant never hearing the words "We would like you to go see a specialist." At those words, our hearts grew heavy. As first-time parents, we didn't know what to expect. Thoughts of which onesie would be cutest on our baby turned to which doctor we should see for the questions we had.

Prenatal care seems to consist of a multitude of rotating doctors and nurses who fill in for one another on a daily basis, and seeing a perinatal specialist was no different. We were always hopeful that whoever stepped into our room would give us uplifting news. You almost wish they would lie to you for a split second, just to give you some comfort, but they don't. Test results and diagnoses flew through the air, hitting us like bullets in our hearts as they told us her chances were no better than the flip of a coin—fifty-fifty. We told ourselves she would be fine, that surely she would survive, and this allowed us to go on. Days and doctor visits piled up as we approached "The Big Day."

Harper's birth was nothing short of hectic, but gazing upon her with welcoming eyes was worth all the confusion and lack of sleep. If I could pinpoint the dumbest thing I ever did as a parent, it would be closing the bar where I worked the night before Harper's birth was scheduled via C-section at 5:30 a.m. But you do what you have to do. I left the bar at 3:24 a.m. to get a pointless hour's sleep, which turned into about fifteen minutes before I awoke to my clock reading 5:07. Realizing the C-section was in twenty minutes, we ran with a handful of what we thought we needed and drove like a bat out of hell to the hospital. I thought it essential to cast Erin out at the mouth of the emergency room, but as I parked the car, I realized that the hospital is like the military—you hurry up to wait.

One of the worst parts of Harper's birth for me was

wearing a god-awful getup that looked like a hazmat suit. I was sweating like a pig in a bacon factory. As we anxiously waited for our slew of doctors to enter the room, text messages came rolling in, making my phone sound like an alarm clock that wouldn't shut up.

"We're ready when you are" were the words that made my head blow up like a balloon and my stomach sink below sea level. We marched into the prep room as Erin was wheeled in. In a million years, nothing could have prepared me for watching a C-section. The birth went by in a blur, though the sight of all that blood and tissue flopping around was mitigated by a beautiful little nugget escaping the wound. Harper levitated not to me or her mommy, but to a respirator—helpless and without a cry. There was no comforting squeal, yelp, or moan—only the sounds of footsteps and the foreign-sounding words of the doctors as they prepped her and took her away to the NICU (the neonatal intensive care unit).

We watched the hours stream by with heavy eyes and halting hearts. No one knew what the outcome of those first twenty-four hours would be. These were some of the most pivotal moments of her life, but unfortunately, not the worst. Watching the clock was pointless; it was nothing more than a decoration on a blank wall. Instead, we kept our eyes focused on the door, waiting for confirmation that we would be able to meet our newborn.

After what seemed like an eternity, the words "You can go back and see her" came tumbling out of the mouth of our nurse. At the NICU, we washed up, suited up, and went inside to meet the most astonishing little angel we had ever encountered: Harper Ann Stanfield. Words melted from my tongue as I became speechless; all I had was laughter and love. At that moment we were a family; we had broken the barriers of uncertainty and fear to be together as one. No feeling will ever compare to that moment.

Hours became minutes and minutes turned to seconds as the time we spent beside Harper's "bed" grew more and more intoxicating. We were both exhausted and knew she must be too, so eventually we left her to rest. That's when things seemed to take a turn for the worse, though really, we were just learning how serious Harper's situation was.

Taking a moment to ourselves, Erin and I were discussing the situation at hand when our neonatologist entered the room.

"We need to transfer her to MCV," he muttered, certain and emotional, as he was a close friend and largely the reason why we'd chosen the hospital we did.

All blood flow stopped, all thoughts died, and our only question was "Why?"

He explained to us what we already knew: that she was potentially going to need extracorporeal membrane oxygenation (ECMO), or essentially life support, something his hospital did not possess. As we watched a team prepare her for transfer, we saw just how vulnerable she was, and how lethal CDH was. Her oxygen saturation levels plummeted, her heart rate sank, and no one in the room breathed easy. Her stats continued to roller coaster until finally, after several attempts, she lay atop the transfer unit. With haste, they wheeled her to the elevator, out the door, and into the ambulance to whisk her away to MCV.

As for Erin and me, feelings of love, pain, stress, and discomfort weighed upon us, as she could not be discharged from the hospital. It was the longest night of our lives. I would be lying if I said I didn't think about sneaking out of Erin's hospital room to visit Harper at MCV, but I knew Erin would need me to maintain her emotional sanity.

When daylight broke and her discharge papers surfaced, we made the mad dash to be at Harper's side. As Murphy's Law would have it, traffic was terrible, and finding our way around the monstrosity of a hospital was like trying to navigate a theme park. Finally, we came to the Fort Knox that was the NICU at MCV. Walking as fast as we could without running, we made a beeline for Harper. As we surrounded her, we were introduced to the staff of nurses and doctors who would eventually come to be like family, and who would feel a profound attachment to our daughter.

Family and friends called, texted, and Facebook messaged, asking questions about how she was doing and what they could do to help us in our time of need. Immediate family would eventually litter the room to gaze upon Harper and give her the nickname TooT, a name thrown out by her grandmother, Carol Adkins, in an effort to capture her adorable nature in one word. We came to realize that this name was too perfect, being that her mother, Erin, was nicknamed Terd . . . classy, I know. As we all came together at Harper's side, many other friends remained in the dark. So, in an effort to keep everyone up to date on her status, I started a Facebook page about Harper's battle (www.facebook.com/CDHernia). In hindsight, it seems fitting that a technology like Facebook would bring Harper so much love and support, as technology and machines would be some of her greatest allies in her trials to come.

Over the next few days, our lives began to revolve around wires, tubes, machines, and Harper . . . our Little TooT. These elements became as much a part of her life as the doctors and nurses did. And while we wished we could just take her home and be rid of the hospital and the constant parade of new names and faces, we knew that those healthcare workers truly cared about Harper. They were each invested in her struggle, almost as if she gravitated others toward her to heal them in some small way. I began to comprehend the inspirational power our tiny daughter possessed— by simple virtue of her will to keep on living.

There are no comforting words I can offer about the pictures and thoughts that you're about to encounter. They aren't meant to shock, only to convey my passion for a love that I hope everyone will one day feel. As you read this book, I want you to think about each post as if you were there with us from the start. Every moment of every hour, you're wondering what will happen next and dreading the answer. Imagine feeling like a criminal awaiting his sentence as you arrive at the hospital each day to hear about the issues troubling your daughter. You never know for sure whether you will be told "She's doing fine" or "There is nothing more we can do." You weigh your options, as if a devil and angel are sitting on each shoulder, only you don't know which is which. Just as we chose to keep going each day, you have the option to keep reading further. Do it for you, for your heart, and maybe for some comfort in your future trials. For what it is worth, even though I do not know you, I love you. Remember that.

Post 1:
Launch: August 23

On April 25th, my girlfriend, Erin Byers, and I went to Henrico Doctors Hospital and affirmed what we already had an idea of—SHE WAS PREGNANT! We couldn't have been happier. A little time went by and we returned to the hospital. Upon visiting the OB/GYN and going through the ultrasound, we were told that our child had a physical disorder, CDH (congenital diaphragmatic hernia). We had no idea what to expect. We were told that a hole in her diaphragm had allowed her stomach and part of her intestines to remain in her chest, impeding the development of her left lung. Our hearts sank; however, we knew we had to stay positive for the baby. Months went by, and finally the day came: August 20, 2012. Erin gave birth by C-section to Harper Ann Stanfield, a beautiful, 7.2-pound, 20-inch angel. From there she was quickly rushed to the NICU, where she remained stable until the following night, when she had to be transferred to MCV hospital, where she remains. Help us raise awareness for future angels with this disorder.

Post 2:
August 23, 1:43 p.m.

My daughter, Harper Ann Stanfield, is suffering from CDH, and I just want to start promoting awareness for this disorder, which has little preventative research being done. She is an angel, and I feel as though maybe I can make a difference in future cases. I love my daughter, so help me gather enough likes to push for a change for future angels.

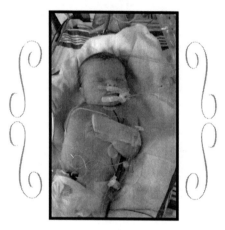

Post 3:
August 23, 2:59 p.m.

As of right now, she is stable. She is stubborn and lowers her vitals when she is bothered. However, she continues to be a fighter. We are on our way to see her and make sure she is still as feisty as always. Tune in to this page for updates, and remember to tell a friend about this page so we can spread the word. For every person who becomes aware of this disorder, we are one step closer to finding a cure!

Post 4:
August 23, 10:11 p.m.

Little TooT (Harper) is doing well as of right now. Her vitals are stable, though we were informed that last night her heart rate sank to 20 beats per minute . . . but she is back up and doing better. Hopefully she can continue to do well all night!

Post 5:
August 24, 11:21 a.m.

Well, we had a good night last night. Harper didn't have any drastic drops in vitals. She is going off of her epinephrine drip (helps with blood pressure) and is awake and lively. She has to be sedated again to keep her little butt from pulling out some wiring!

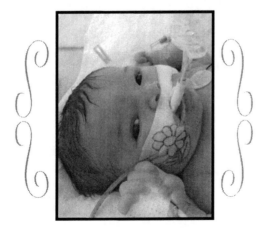

Post 6:
August 24, 11:53 p.m.

So today was a GREAT DAY in the world of Miss Harper! Her sedatives were lowered, and, as you can see from the former post, she has a beautiful little set of eyes. She is getting better with breathing . . . every little bit helps, but she is looking to have surgery sometime next week! Please pray, and hopefully she will keep it up! AND remember to keep sharing this Facebook page and support the fund. Don't feel obligated to donate, but show your support!

Post 7:
August 25, 10:55 p.m.

Well, today was a good day for Miss Harper. She is stable and ACTIVE! Probably more than her daddy wants her to be, but I doubt she cares. :P

Post 8:
August 26, 1:06 a.m.

"Off to bed," she said. Goodnight Little TooT!

> Comment from Haley Cash: I was born with a diaphragmatic hernia and am 28 years old. Thought it was a crazy coincidence that a friend of mine "liked" your page. You all will be in my thoughts. Keep your heads high and love that baby with everything you have!

Post 9:
August 26, 1:25 p.m.

We had a little bit of a rough night last night. Vitals went down, but the neonatologist says it isn't a "setback," so they are still thinking surgery next week. She needs to let the doctors help, but she does what she wants and tries to do her own thing . . . I'd say she got her mom's stubborn gene . . . :P

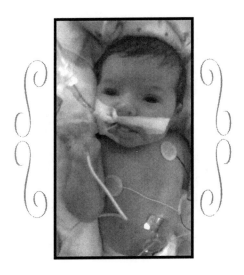

Post 10:
August 26, 3:09 p.m.

Unfortunately they are saying to cut down on nighttime visiting . . . so NO visiting after 8 P.M. I will miss kissing her goodnight. :(@CDH_Help

Post 11:
August 27, 2:11 p.m.

Baby Harper is struggling . . . her stats went down, and she is being prepared for the last resort ECMO. I will keep you posted. Pray. @CDH_Help

Post 12:
August 27, 3:08 p.m.

Harper is minutes before going for EMCO. Got to get those heart and lungs strong for the corrective surgery! You can make it, little one. It's not a last resort; it's a fresh start!

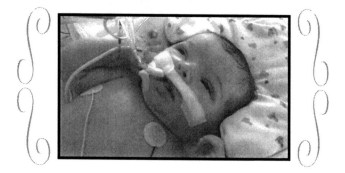

Post 13:
August 27, 8:00 p.m.

She made it onto ECMO, and her vitals are stable. The next 24 hours are critical, but she is quite the trooper, and we have a lot of people cheering her on and a lot of angels looking down upon her . . .

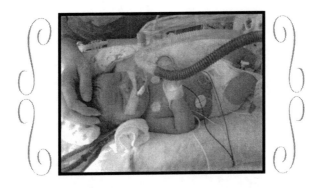

Comment from Danny Byers: Be strong, little
sweetheart. Grandpa loves you and is praying for you.

Post 14:
August 28, 11:59 p.m.

Miss Harper had a better day today. Her vitals are
staying up, and evidently she doesn't like being tickled
(sorry, Daddy loves you). I just want to tell everyone
thank you for all your prayers and for being there for
Harper in her time of need. She will pull through. I
know it!

Post 15:
August 29, 2:10 p.m.

Little Miss TooT had a great night last night; she is
active and now has a little glowing hand and toe . . .
E.T. phone home!* Hopefully sooner rather than later
she will be able to come home!

*The glowing was due to the pulse oximeter wrapped around
her hand and toe, which monitored her oxygen saturation
levels.*

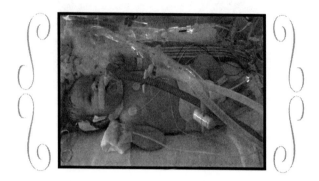

Post 16:
August 30, 2:03 p.m.

Just a quick update! Harper is doing better today! She was a bit too active and needed to calm those little hands and feet, so a heavier sedative was given, but she is doing better and her lung conditioning starts today! I hope she can battle further and get home to her mommy and daddy!

> Comment from Debbie Dye: Made our morning a lot better. Keep up the good work, Harper. Love you all!

Post 17:
August 30, 8:43 p.m.

Miss Harper telling Momma hello and feeling good as she does her lung conditioning and weans herself off of ECMO, or the heart/lung bypass . . . she looks beautiful. :)

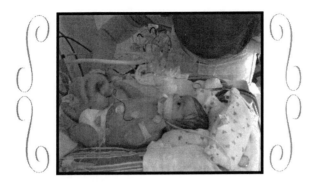

Post 18:
August 31, 2:10 p.m.

Well, Harper had a good night and morning. She did have to have a bolus (basically a sedative) to calm her little butt down, although as you can see in the picture, she has no problem holding on to Momma! :) Today is day 2 for lung conditioning, and we are hoping she can progress forward! Thanks again to everyone for your support!

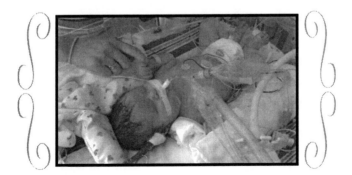

Post 19:
August 31, 9:46 p.m.

It seems as though there are more and more machines every time we arrive. It is a scary thing to see, but I have to keep in mind that every machine is helping my child push forward, and no matter how crowded and intimidating they look, they are all necessary. I call it her space shuttle. :)

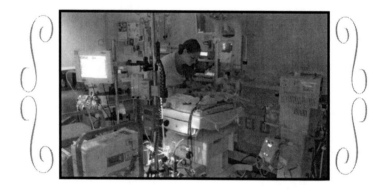

Post 20:
September 1, 7:47 p.m.

So this is a look at Miss Harper from the inside. Her lung conditioning is going great! The black on the left X-ray is bowel and some lung at 8 a.m. this morning . . . the one on the right is her at 5 p.m. The lung progression is great! All of the dark is air in the lungs, and yes, there is still bowel in the chest, but she is doing very well today!

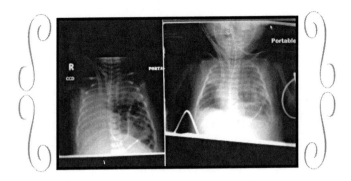

Post 21:
September 2, 3:10 p.m.

She already gives me that look of "Who the hell do you think you are?" Got to love that, haha. Today she is doing okay. We had a trial run without ECMO, which didn't go well . . . but one day at a time. We will get there. They are saying there is a possibility of surgery on ECMO, which is not what we want, but I have faith that she will make it!

Post 22:
September 3, 4:11 a.m.

So today was a slight setback . . . She has less air in her lungs and a lot of pulmonary hypertension (blood avoiding the lungs); however, that may be because she had an obstruction in her airway (mucus). They think that she may do better throughout the night and into tomorrow. She is still fighting, and I know in my heart that with the support that you all are giving, she will prevail. Remember, keep letting people know about our Facebook page and Help Harper Head Home!

Post 23:
September 3, 4:31 a.m.

Amanda Hollandsworth has a child facing open-heart surgery and asked me if I would promote her page, and I told her I would be obliged to do so, because in the end, it is not about me, or any of us; it is about the children we together can help.

Post 24:
September 3, 12:29 p.m.

Melanie Braun brought this child to my attention, and she needs a bit of help as well, so check out her page and remember, every bit of support you give can change a child's life!

Post 25:
September 3, 1:48 p.m.

Today is a bit better in the world of Miss Harper. As I posted yesterday, she had a bit of a rough day internally, but today we are seeing signs of improvement. Her vitals are solid, and she is back on track with being active! Here is a picture after Daddy tickled her. Harper is looking at Mommy and saying with her eyes, "Why did you bring him?" :)

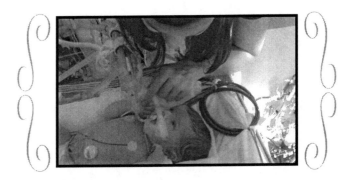

Post 26:
September 4, 1:39 a.m.

Today was an up-and-down roller coaster, but ultimately it was a good day. Harper boded well for the most part, and all we can do is sit back and pray!

Post 27:
September 4, 7:34 p.m.

Today was a busy day for our Little TooT. She was given antibiotics to fight possible pneumonia. But we also found that her lungs are somewhat more developed than previously anticipated after her "bronc" (a camera put down her throat to observe the inside of her lungs) so that is a definite plus! However, today we found out that a beautiful little guy has passed away—Liam Lyon, born with half of a heart—so this post is for him. We can only hope that is he watching and helping our little angel through her battle.

Post 28:
September 5, 3:22 p.m.

We got some bad news today. We were told that her right lung (the healthier lung) is not responding to the change from ventilator to oscillator and is having difficulty reopening on a normal oscillator. We are in the process of switching her to a conventional ventilator, which will hopefully open up that lung. If she cannot open up that right lung by Monday, we are looking at surgery on ECMO by next Wednesday, which has a higher risk of bleeding out than surgery without it. Kyle, our nurse at the MCV NICU, is hopeful, and we know she can hang in there!

Post 29:
September 5, 4:35 p.m.

Well, Harper has been switched from the oscillator to a more normal breathing machine. So instead of a ton of tiny breaths per minute, she will be taking about 30 normal breaths per minute. They did this in hopes of opening up that right lung. We'll get an X-ray in an hour or so to check the status of her progress. It's been a very busy day today for Little TooT.

Post 30:
September 5, 9:55 p.m.

I just want to give my regards and thoughts to Ian Mortensen and his son Isaac, who has cerebral palsy.

I'll be thinking about you, man, and I hope to one day have Harper meet Isaac!

Post 31:
September 6, 4:57 p.m.

I figured you all would like to see some of what goes on in the NICU room, so I posted this video* I took. She is doing much better. Her second trial run off EMCO was better, and her X-rays looked much better as well! Tell me what you think of keeping the occasional video feed coming.

The video displayed an everyday walk around Harper's room, including the washing-up process and a more in-depth look at the machinery used to keep Harper alive.

Post 32:
September 7, 1:53 p.m.

It was a hard-working morning for TooT! The doctors clamped off the ECMO to test her ability to stabilize on an oscillator alone. She did okay. She had an echocardiogram (echo) to see how her heart reacted, which went well, but she is still on ECMO. Monday is the deadline before she has to go into surgery on ECMO. Pray hard and think happy thoughts. Come on, Shorty!

Post 33:
September 8, 1:36 p.m.

Even though our journey is not over, I just wanted to take a minute to thank each and every one of you who has helped us through prayer, thoughts, and donations. I was sitting here looking through each post, astonished and proud of how Harper has impacted so many lives. You all have made us stronger. You are all family in our eyes, and I hope Harper will one day know just how many people were there for her in her time of need. Thank you all. :)

Post 34:
September 8, 6:31 p.m.

Harper says "Hi" to everyone and hopes you are all doing well! She has had a busy day today. Got her dressing changed on her neck and had some sedations; HOWEVER, the big news is that her surgery is being pushed up to Monday the 10th of September. She will be on ECMO, but she is becoming dependent on the machine and we cannot have that . . . so this is big news and scary news, but she doesn't seem to care, she's being a big goofball!

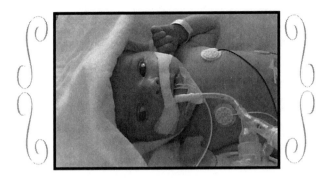

Post 35:
September 9, 12:14 p.m.

Jaden's mommy just contacted me and asked me to help spread the word for her little guy, I hope this helps! He looks like a strong little man!*

Jaden suffered from hydranencephaly, a rare disorder of the brain where the cerebral hemispheres are absent and cerebrospinal fluid sacs reside there instead.

Post 36:
September 9, 12:43 p.m.

Harper has been moved to the procedure room and has been prepped for surgery tomorrow morning at about 8 a.m. She seems to be doing okay, other than a little bit of high blood pressure due to the move. She did fine. Our Little TooT is being brave!

Post 37:
September 10, 12:01 p.m.

Little miss fancy pants with her pinky up. :) Tomorrow is the big day. Her corrective surgery is happening early in the morning. We're staying positive and leaving it in God's hands.

> And though she be but little, she is fierce.
>
> —William Shakespeare

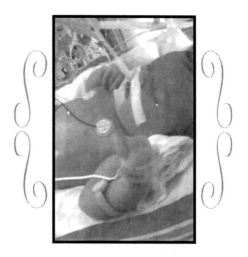

Post 38:
September 10, 6:27 p.m.

Ella's Auntie Tammy asked me to post about her niece, who had a stroke, and as you know I never mind helping a child with thoughts and prayers for a safe journey!

Post 39:
September 10, 8:11 a.m.

She is in surgery now. This is just a quick video of the room and doctors prepping the room. Please pray for her; she is our Little TooT, and she needs all of you now more than ever. Thank you from the bottom of our hearts for being there for us in our time of need. We love you all.

Post 40:
September 10, 11:11 a.m.

Here is what we know: the surgery went fine, she is swollen and partially still open, as there were fluids coming out. She is bleeding from an unknown source at this time. She is stable, and a patch was put on her diaphragm. It paints an uneasy picture, but we are hopeful. I promise you will know more as we find more things out. Again, thank you all for your support.

Post 41:
September 10, 12:05 p.m.

She is losing a lot of blood at a rapid rate, and she has heightened to a more critical level . . . please pray for my baby.

Post 42:
September 10, 1:08 p.m.

Thank you, Nikki,* and thank all of you for your prayers. We just saw her, and in my eyes, even with all that is going on after surgery, she is still the most beautiful thing in the world . . .

> *Nikki had a renowned blog with thousands of followers. She wrote a post about Harper and how her journey had made her reflect on life in new ways.*

Post 43:
September 10, 2:40 p.m.

Combined with surgery, Harper has lost over 500 cc of blood; the normal baby has only about 240 cc of blood in their body. The doctors are pumping in 80 cc every hour at least. She is in critical condition and is unstable. They cannot close the wound because of excess swelling in her abdomen. I will keep you updated. It is truly remarkable, though: she still looks like an angel even in her current state . . .

Post 44:
September 10, 4:52 p.m.

I have been reading your posts all day as I sit in the waiting room hoping to hear about Harper's status. We just got an update: She is still in critical condition and they are giving her more platelets and blood clotting medicine, but she has not yet responded to other treatments. They fear that when they suture the wound it will re-aggravate the bleeding, but it has to be done. Please share this page so I can continue to read these posts, as it will be a long night and Harper needs all the encouragement she can get. In my eyes, you are all family. Thank you, and we love you all.

Post 45:
September 10, 7:35 p.m.

They have gone back into surgery to try to stop the bleeding, but as of last, they had not found the source. Surgery is still in progress . . . hang in there, baby girl . . .

Post 46:
September 10, 10:10 p.m.

As of right now, they have controlled the bleeding. Harper, however, has a long road to go. The bleeding was due to openings in a few blood vessels around her ribs, as the ribs were anchoring the sutures for the patch on her diaphragm. They had to cut that patch and go into her chest, as there was a lot of blood. Now they have gauze in place, essentially soaking the blood and holding her organs, etc. in place. She did well through surgery and has more surgery to go through, so as of right now, her bleeding has gone down significantly, but she is still in a critical state. She is a fighter and I am so proud of how well she is standing her ground. I love you, Harper, more than you can ever imagine . . .

Post 47:
September 10, 11:24 p.m.

Harper is defying so many odds . . . do you believe in miracles? Answer and share this if you do.*

834 people answered yes.

Post 48:
September 11, 10:24 a.m.

I wish I had better things to tell you all this morning, but I don't . . . Harper has got another surgical battle on her hands. She is very swollen throughout her body today, the acidity in her blood is high and needs to be lowered, and the gauze pads are being replaced. The good thing is there is no imminent bleeding. However, the ECMO circuit has to be replaced, potentially setting her back . . . We are also being told that she may have signs of ischemia in the bowel, which may or may not be dead bowel. She is in surgery now. Please pray and keep others up-to-date and share . . .

Post 49:
September 11, 12:57 p.m.

So Harper is struggling . . . She has gone back to bleeding more, 135 cc in the past hour; however, it is not as much as it was yesterday. She has to be put on a medicine called Factor-7. Factor-7 helps to clot bleeding, however, it risks causing clotting in all different areas of the body, both extremities and organs, therefore there is the risk of losing areas of the body to blood clots. She is also being put on a new ECMO circuit, which—with her being open from surgery and after so much stress on her system with Factor-7, etc.—gives her a 50-50 shot of making it through the transition. Harper, be strong baby, Mommy and Daddy and everyone here loves you . . . be strong . . .

Post 50:
September 11, 3:55 p.m.

She is presently defying odds again! For now she is doing well with the Factor-7 . . . for now. She did well on the ECMO circuit transfer (during that 3-minute period she did well only on the oscillator). Harper is extremely swollen right now, though, and there is a downside: her kidneys are failing for the time being, and there is talk of dialysis, which is a scary thought. She has continued to bleed excessively, which has been hard on her kidneys. So, as we prayed before, we pray now: Please stop bleeding, Little TooT, and let's push forward. :) Again, please, please SHARE this post and get more people and prayers flowing. It seems to be working little by little . . .

Post 51:
September 11, 5:04 p.m.

As I sit and stand and pace and look at every opening of that waiting room door, yearning for an update on how Little TooT is doing, I constantly get reminders of how much Harper is loved by reading the posts, prayers, and messages you all have sent, and I realize how lucky I am to have people like you following, but also how lucky Harper is to have so many people who care. I can't not recognize the date that is upon us and how 11 years ago, many men, women, and children did not have the chance to fight back, but lost their lives in a tragedy that will live in our hearts forever, and for that, Harper, Erin, our family, and I send a prayer back to all of the families who lost loved ones. May they watch over you . . . and may you share this so that it may commemorate them . . .

Post 52:
September 11, 10:09 p.m.

As of right now, Harper has all but stopped excessive bleeding! She has evened out her blood pressure medications, and while she does have another surgery to go through, we were told to report from the nurses, "As far as all things considered, she has had a good afternoon." They will wait and let her stabilize for a bit before her next surgery, but as of right now, we are all smiles. We are still preparing for another big battle, but Harper is defying the odds! Please share this, as every prayer has been helping, and we need to stockpile the prayers for Harper's battle to come!

24

Post 53:
September 12, 10:33 a.m.

Good morning, all. Today will be a more interactive day with Harper's momma, as I, her daddy (the one who does most of the posting), will have to go to work at 5 p.m. tonight. Obviously I want to be by her side, but unfortunately, as I told you all before, bills have to be paid to give Harper the life she deserves. So be good to Little TooT's momma (Terd :P)! Harper had an okay night . . . she did bleed some more, but again, it is getting less and less. She is a fighter and a wiggler, so they had to go up on sedation as she is still open. She is still peeing, which means those kidneys are working! Surgery will be halted today, as she has had a rough few days and Miss TooT needs to heal up before they can go back in. Stay tuned for more updates, and remember to keep sharing. We can always use more prayers for our little angel!

Post 54:
September 12, 12:28 p.m.

This is Daddy . . . I will be at my daughter's side all day and night as we have just found out that she has taken a turn for the worse and the doctors do not know if she will make it . . . we just had the discussion as to whether we should try surgery one more time or let nature take its course and put our angel to rest. As I sit here typing, crying, and longing to hold my child, I can't help but read the prayers you all have sent us over these days and weeks . . . I want so bad to personally thank every one of you in person with Harper in my arms, but I don't know if that will ever happen. I love you all, as does Erin, and most of all Harper . . .

Post 55:
September 12, 3:07 p.m.

We have elected to go for one more shot, and she is being prepped for surgery now . . . I couldn't give in to letting her go without one more shot. I love you, angel, be strong. You are stronger than us all. I will let you all know how surgery goes. Share for prayers . . . we love you all.

Post 56:
September 12, 4:49 p.m.

So, we got an update . . . They are still in surgery and found some bleeding around the spleen, but they are not certain that the spleen is the source of the bleeding. Her right lung is being compressed by swelling, so a pigtail catheter is being placed to help drain the fluid from all of the swelling. We will keep you posted. As always, share for prayer . . .

Post 57:
September 12, 6:53 p.m.

We have an update . . . She is out of surgery, and they

found what they think was a major source of bleeding on the spleen, where some tissue attached to the exterior of the spleen was torn. It's miraculous that she has endured all four surgeries. What is even more incredible is that she was taken off of ECMO (her life support system that takes deoxygenated blood out of her system and replaces it with oxygenated blood through the artery in her neck) and held her own for 10 minutes! They placed the catheter in her right chest cavity to drain fluid. We've been told that her mortality risk is high, but, as her surgeon said, "It is a miracle she's still with us." So we're hoping for another miracle. She won't give up or give in! But these next few hours are critical. Share for prayer, and donate if you can! We love you all, and you are continuing to give Harper strength, so we thank you a million times over!

Post 58:
September 12, 9:00 p.m.

Harper is stable for the time being. She still has a hard road ahead, and we will keep you updated if anything changes!

Post 59:
September 13, 12:30 a.m.

Positive news for baby Harper! Harper has not had to have her dressings changed in over 3 hours, which means much of the bleeding has been reduced. She is peeing a little bit more and her lactate levels are down.

This means her cells are at less risk of dying, causing loss of limbs, organs, etc. (her lactate levels are at 1.7 and were at 16 yesterday!). She still has oozing (a mixture of bleeding and other bodily secretions) coming from her chest, but it too has reduced! Overall, she is looking much better than yesterday! The doctors and nurses still want us to be aware that she is in a very critical state, but she IS looking better!

Post 60:
September 13, 10:46 a.m.

An update . . . Harper's dressing was changed at 3 a.m., and she had lost 75 cc, so there was a bit of bleeding; however, it has not been changed since then, which is huge! Her dopamine levels went up, which means she needs a little bit of help for her blood pressure. She's urinating normally, and they are pulling a lot of fluid out of her, which calms down a lot of that swelling! The odds tell us she shouldn't even be alive, but Harper is defying those odds and pushing forward . . . and winning right now! Daddy is about to cry he is so happy! :) Remember, share for prayer, and Help Harper Head Home!

Post 61:
September 13, 1:38 p.m.

While I know some of you may not want to see her close up, as it can be unsettling, I wanted to let you all see a more tasteful photo of how Little TooT is looking and handling the surgery and ECMO. She is doing as well as well as can be expected right now. As always, share for prayer! She couldn't have done this without y'all!

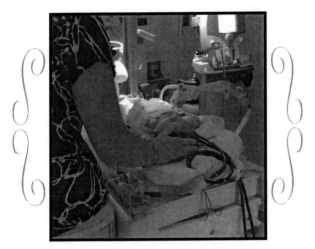

Post 62:
September 13, 2:34 p.m.

As this page is about Harper's struggle with CDH, I want to remind everyone that there are other angels out there with the same condition. CDH affects 1,600 children in the U.S. every year, so awareness is key, and spreading the word is crucial! I want to know if you have any suggestions for how to spread awareness for these innocent children. Any suggestion is a good suggestion! I have been so impressed with the sharing. Keep it up, and let's get all CDH children home! Harper also squeezed my finger, and it made me tear up a bit. She knows she has so much love around her! :)

Post 63:
September 13, 3:43 p.m.

Earlier we received a request to show a picture of Harper up close, so here it is. As parents, we can see past the bandages and tubes to see what a beautiful angel Harper really is, and I hope others can as well. She is swollen but doing much better today than she was at this time yesterday. They have told us that she will have several more surgeries before she is repaired, but she has to show she is strong enough to be off of ECMO to move further. The bleeding has lowered, and her urine output has increased. They have lowered her clotting medications to allow her body to try to do it on its own. Even through the wiring and tubes, she is still absolutely gorgeous . . .

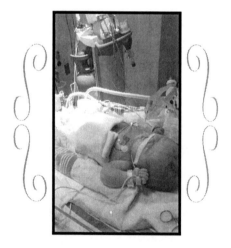

Post 64:
September 13, 5:53 p.m.

They are currently working on increasing her blood pressure to be able to take off more fluid around her body, so she is being put back on epinephrine (adrenaline, basically). This can be a good thing and a bad thing. If they take too much off, it could make her blood pressure plummet; however, it was comforting to see her look at me as I kissed her on the forehead. Stay strong, baby girl! We all love you! Share for prayer; she needs her strength for this!

Post 65:
September 13, 9:32 p.m.

Tonight we discussed with the nurses, doctors, and respiratory therapists how they have never witnessed anything like this . . . not just Harper's miracles, but how a family and so many people have come together to witness what they say they thought to be "impossible." It's amazing to see a newborn with such huge odds against her fighting for her life and breaking down so many barriers to get back to looking at her mommy, daddy, grandparents, aunts, and uncles. Harper is doing better as every hour passes now. We know she will keep her fight through future surgery. Tonight, this post is for all of you out there who have prayed and helped bring my angel's eyes back to me. Thank you, and I love you all.

Post 66:
September 14, 11:20 a.m.

So it will be a busy day for Miss Harper today. She has to have all dressings replaced on her open abdominal wound and on her neck, where the ECMO machine is entering. The dressing on her abdomen is the one to be more worried about, as the last time they changed it, she bled out due to raw organs and easily torn tissues. So this is something I will be focusing on. She has stopped receiving a constant flow of blood and is given more as needed, which is a good sign. However, with the dressing changes, etc., that could change. Also, with the blood pooling under her body, it has caused her skin to become raw on her back and butt . . . so they are having people come in to deal with that, and to see if she can be placed in a more comfortable position. All in all, it may be another roller coaster day for Little TooT . . . Please pray that she stays strong today. I will keep everyone updated on how she does after each change. As always, share for a prayer and Help Harper Head Home . . .

Post 67:
September 14, 1:30 p.m.

We just talked with the surgeon about the dressing changes, and she did great! She is awake and alert; however, repair of the diaphragm may not happen for months. She has had such a rough past couple of days that they do not feel comfortable going back in. She will have time to become stronger and bigger, making the issue of bleeding out less likely. They also want to wean her off the ECMO circuit, to help her become self-sustainable. It worries me that she will not be fixed for so long, as there will be days when I'll only be able to see her for short periods of time due to money issues and job musts. After all of the ups and downs, I feel like this is going to bother me the most, and I don't know what to do . . .

Post 68:
September 14, 2:30 p.m.

This video* allows you to see what I, Daddy, see from day to day. We hope this shows a more hands-on experience and helps everyone connect better with us, and most of all Harper.

> *The video depicted the day-to-day daunting tasks we had to go through just to lay our hands upon the forehead of our child: washing our hands from elbow to fingertip, asking permission to enter the NICU, the long walk down the hallway filled with angels fighting for their lives, and finally entering the room littered with machines, lights, and doctors, all of which we blocked out to focus only on Harper, the most beautiful sight to our tired eyes.

Post 69:
September 14, 7:29 p.m.

An update . . . Little TooT is doing okay . . . The doctors have had to increase her dopamine for her blood pressure and she has gotten a saline bolus to calm her little butt down. They are trying to calm down the swelling, and it's working! She is being weaned off the ECMO still, a little at a time. A good note: her X-ray looked much better; she is getting a lot of air into her right lung. However, she still has her left lung compressed, which means that the right lung had better compensate! Overall, she remains in critical condition, but she is doing better! We also wanted to say thank you to some of the people who have come by to show support, and for the goodies! As always, share for prayer; your prayers are working and now some local news stations may want to do a story on our TooT!

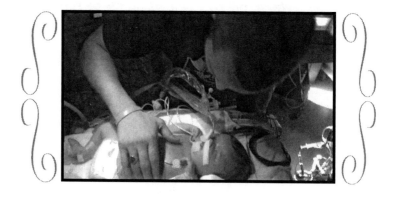

Post 70:
September 15, 12:55 a.m.

As I sit here and scroll one by one through each photo, I think about how lucky I am to be a father to such a wonderful and inspirational angel. She has not only changed my life but the lives of Erin, our families, and most of you all . . . She has shown us all what it takes to be strong and most of all what it takes to prevail . . . She has taught us all more than we could ever teach her about bravery and I cannot thank her enough . . . I love you, TooT . . .

Post 71:
September 15, 11:07 a.m.

Since Little TooT is sleeping, I want to take some time to get to know all of you and your children! As Mommy and I sit here, we would like to see your little ones! Upload a picture and tag yourself in it! We would love to see your family and little toots!

Post 72:
September 15, 12:33 p.m.

Your pictures are making us laugh and smile, and giving us hope for the future. Hopefully we will get to show you all some cute and goofy pictures of TooT in the months and years to come! Keep them coming, and don't forget to tag yourself and your little angel!

Post 73:
September 15, 12:56 p.m.

Just thought I would put a picture up of me when I was little. I think TooT sort of looks a little like me. :)

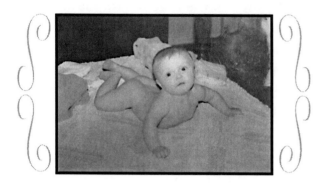

Post 74:
September 15, 1:43 p.m.

This is an exclusive video of something we do not normally get to see: Little TooT waking up! Remember, S4P (Share For Prayer) and a new one . . . R4T (Root For TooT).

Post 75:
September 15, 9:03 p.m.

Well, today has been a rather boring day . . . which is a good thing. Harper has been pretty awake and alert for most of the day, checking everything out. She showed her feisty side earlier by kicking off the bandage around the arterial line in her foot . . . they tried re-taping it, but she obviously did more damage than they thought, as the whole line came out. So now they will no longer be able to monitor her blood pressure continuously or draw blood to run tests on. But luckily they can do all that with a blood pressure cuff and the ECMO machine.

Harper

I (Mommy) have been looking through all of the pics you guys have been posting while sitting in TooT's room today. It has kept me entertained, and I must say, you all have some beautiful little angels! Keep posting them! As always, R4T & S4P.

Post 76:
September 16, 11:15 a.m.

So this morning has been relatively calm; however, she has developed jaundice due to her medication and its effect on her liver, which is due to her TPN, or electrolytes. She has had minimal bleeding, but the doctors have had to up her bolus (sedation) because of yesterday's incident with the line coming out of her foot. She is getting a little more swollen, as they have to pump more fluid into her to try to combat the jaundice, and she has had to have more blood and platelets put in. She is one tough cookie, and we hope that she continues to be a thorn in the side of this disorder! Never forget to S4P and R4T!

Post 77:
September 16, 1:49 p.m.

TooT is hanging in there still. Leslie, her nurse, wants to keep her boring and "super normal" . . . thankfully! Little TooT is now taking all of her medication intravenously because she sprung a leak on her normal medication tubing. Today has not been a hard day on TooT, but it has been a hard day on her momma. I am connecting with many of you on here, and I feel as though I do

not know what to do to make Erin feel better about the situation. It is very difficult to be by Harper's side all of the time from the minute she wakes up to the minute she leaves for bed, and it is taking its toll on her. I cannot tell you how difficult it is to see your child for weeks on end and not be able to hold, hug, and coddle your beautiful newborn. It is an urge that I get every day I see Harper. We long and hope that maybe today will be the day she can be wrapped in our arms. I am trying to stay strong for both of my girls, and I know I can do it if I stay positive. Do any of you have any ideas on how to help with the situation? Any ideas to help her release some stress? Please pray for Harper and her momma. Leave me out of this one—they need it now more than I do. As always S4P, R4T, and please, if you can, donate . . .
Love always,
Daddy

Post 78:
September 16, 8:22 p.m.

Since Daddy put his baby picture up, I thought I might put one up of me (Mommy). More to come, I promise. :)

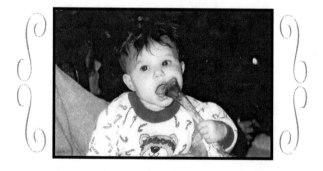

Post 79:
September 16, 9:27 p.m.

Harper had another good night; they gave her blood products because she needed platelets for clotting. She was peeing a little less, because she has been losing fluids, and the swelling is reducing, which is good. However, tomorrow we will likely find out more about where she stands in regard to future surgeries, etc., which will be nerve-wracking! Watch as TooT tells her momma off! Not Daddy though. ;)

Post 80:
September 17, 11:39 a.m.

This morning on TooT! HAPPY 4 WEEKS, TOOT! So . . . they have continued to give her platelets for clotting, but her pee output has slowed down a lot, and they think it may be due to fluid loss. The BIG news . . . they are thinking that they will perform a clamp-off on her ECMO tomorrow to see how she does (basically cut off her life support for a short period to wean her). The plan will be to try and take her off of ECMO by the end of this week. The danger is that if she needs to go back on ECMO after her surgery to fix the hole in her diaphragm, putting her back on will be difficult, as they will have tied off the artery in the right side of her neck. This is all so nerve-wracking, but TooT is always as cool as the other side of the pillow . . . I wish Mommy and Daddy could learn from her. :P

Post 81:
September 17, 5:23 p.m.

S4P, R4T, and donate to help TooT! So TooT had a bit of a tantrum during her changing and her vital checks, which caused her blood pressure to go a bit up, but they got that settled. Now it has gone a bit down, which they think could be attributed to the loss of fluid. She will be getting an echo (looking at her heart) tomorrow before the clamping of her ECMO (life support), which is big, since she hasn't had an echo in a while what with all of the swelling. Otherwise, she is looking pretty good. She just needs to control her emotions with all of the blood pressure stuff. Also, there will be a local station broadcasting in our future for TooT. :)

Post 82:
September 17, 8:42 p.m.

They say that when you become a parent you see things differently and feel things you never thought possible. Watching the nurses change the dressing on Harper's wounds and seeing the soft tears run down her chubby cheeks got to me as I never thought it would. I wasn't mad or outraged that she was uncomfortable or in pain physically. It was the exhaustion and emotional distress exuding from her eyes as she lay there, open and in tears. I wanted nothing more than to assure her it would be okay, and that sooner than later it would be all over. I wanted to hold her and put her head atop

of my shoulder and just say, "Shhh, it's all right," but I can't. It's amazing, the bond that has grown between us and the love I have for her . . . and yet I feel like I barely know her and all she has to offer. But I can't wait to be by her side and hold her every step of the way . . .
Daddy

Post 83:
September 18, 11:02 a.m.

Good morning! Mommy here. It's a big day for Miss TooT: at 2 they will be doing a clamp off from ECMO for about 15-20 minutes. During this time, they will be running blood gases and an echo to monitor her. They said that if all goes as planned, they would like to try to get her off ECMO as early as tomorrow (scary thought!). Keep your fingers crossed that she does well today. They were able to wean her down to a lower level of dopamine administration over the past few days, and her blood pressure seems to be doing all right. Also, Little TooT has been speaking to us here lately; due to a slight leak around her breathing tube, when she opens her mouth, it makes a cute squeaky sound. It's always at different pitches and comes out either really loud or as a soft hum. We can always tell when she's mad or awake and moving around from the noises she makes . . . but today they went ahead and replaced the breathing tube with a bigger one, so no more squeaky TooT. :/
As always, S4P & R4T!

Post 84:
September 18, 4:00 p.m.

Afternoon all, Mommy again. Well, Harper had her clamp off earlier, as planned. She did okay, but nothing that showed she was ready to come off. Her blood pressure stayed at a good level the entire time, but her heart rate and oxygen levels dropped. I could tell she was agitated, but the doctors didn't want to give her anything to calm her down, thinking it might affect the readings they were getting. Luckily, she did better than the last time they tried. They have planned for another run tomorrow but with different factors in play. They also decided to switch her ventilator again, back to the conventional one, to see what it does, since her right lung is fully expanded. The X-ray should be coming back soon to tell us if it will work or not. Thank you all for the prayers this afternoon! As always, S4P & R4T.

Post 85:
September 18, 10:35 p.m.

This is Daddy. Today was one of the more difficult days I have had as a father. Yesterday it was watching the dressing change . . . today it was the absence . . . Watching . . . waiting . . . the seconds, minutes, and hours rolled by as I paced around at work, knowing Harper was being prepped for a struggle. I hated the feeling of not being by her side, and a pit grew in my stomach, followed by a lump in my throat as

I waited for a phone call to tell me everything was okay. However, I didn't get that phone call. The phone murmured, "She only lasted 8 minutes off of ECMO and struggled." My heart fell. It was a feeling of overwhelming heartbreak and angst. As the blood rushed out of my face and my co-workers asked, "Is everything okay?" all I could think was, "Why wasn't I at her side?" I called and got a dear co-worker and friend to come in and help me get away. He was speedy, but minutes seemed to turn into days and hours into years as I waited until I could race to the hospital to give TooT a kiss and say, "I'm here, sweet pea . . . " I wish that feeling on no one. Goodnight. Harper is resting for tomorrow. She clamps out at 9 a.m. . . . We will keep you all up to date. As always, S4P, R4T, and donate to Help Harper Head Home.

Post 86:
September 19, 10:16 a.m.

Daddy again . . . This morning TooT got to strut her stuff. The clamping began today at 9:31 a.m. As Mommy and I and a slew of nurses, respiratory therapists, doctors, attendees, and whoever else stood watching and trying not to faint, TooT did her thing. She was on full support, which is not the best scenario, but she withstood longer off of ECMO than anticipated. We all began to smile as she approached the 15-minute mark. She did better than anyone had imagined. It was almost as if she were telling us, "Watch this!" And we did. Who knew a TooT could be so strong? Tomorrow we try with less help, and more TooT strength . . .

Post 87:
September 19, 3:05 p.m.

Daddy here . . . We did the interview with CBS News, and it was like walking step by step down the path we've gotten to know so well. Pain, heartache, strength, love, happiness . . . It was a recap of every emotion and memory we've experienced on this roller coaster journey. Upon finishing the interview, we raced back to the hospital, prepared to be inundated with changes and vital stats—only to find the nurses calm and relaxed, and TooT exuding the same. It was a weird feeling. Everything seemed so at ease, and for the first time, even TooT's "cry-face" was not enough to bother me. Erin looked at me, and I at her, and with a loving feeling, we calmed Harper as parents. We were engulfed in a sense of family . . .

Post 88:
September 19, 3:24 p.m.

The CBS interview will air tonight on the 6 o'clock news on Channel 6 for you local Richmonders; we will be putting the link up as well for everyone else! Thanks for everything, and we love you all (TooT is shaking her arm to wave at you right now)! :)

Post 89:
September 19, 6:39 p.m.

Please stop by Layne's* page and support his journey!
Good luck, Layne. We will all be praying!

> * Layne was born with hypoplastic left heart syndrome (HLHS),
> a very rare congenital heart defect in which the left ventricle of
> the heart is extremely underdeveloped.

Post 90:
September 19, 9:17 p.m.

CBS will be airing the story again tonight at 11 p.m.
and again tomorrow morning. They also played it at 6
p.m. and 7 p.m. earlier tonight, which as Tracy Sears
(the reporter) stated, "is unheard of."
Harper is currently receiving antibiotics for a possible
infection—nothing detrimental—so she is sleeping
tight; however her story is not . . . Enjoy. It made us
smile and cry! :)
As always, S4P, R4T, and donate if you can. :)

Post 91:
September 19, 11:59 p.m.

As always, I will share for a family in need. Go by their
page and help Team Peluso!*

> *The Pelusos are a family that unfortunately had to endure the
> loss of three children to various factors and were reaching out
> for support.

Post 92:
September 20, 10:09 a.m.

Running, racing, traffic frustration, and a sense of sheer unsettling panic . . . these were the obstacles that stood in our way as we journeyed to the NICU after what seemed like an eternal much-needed slumber. We arrived in the labyrinth of a parking deck to find that parking was plagued by Murphy's Law and a painfully lethargic driver taking his time. As we parked in what seemed to be a space for a clown car, we jumped out and ran to the elevator to ascend to the hospital ground floor. Speed walking (so as to not freak out any guard by running), we took the last remaining awkward, doctor-filled elevator to the NICU, washed for what seemed like days, and made a beeline for Harper. "Excuse me!" was the phrase of the hour as we made our way inside the room to hear "She is doing well at 9 minutes on the ECMO clamping." Smiles of utter relief and joy filled the room as Mommy and I giggled in a calm. 10, 11, 12 . . . The minutes kept going, and blood gas levels kept rolling off the doctor's tongue as if to sound off a march. Finally, 15—she had done it! Harper defied the odds, and in less than one week, she had gone from knocking on Heaven's door to making the doctors believe in miracles . . . Harper will be taken off of ECMO later this afternoon, which will be scary in and of itself, but I have faith that this TooT is not afraid of even the most daunting of tasks!

Post 93:
September 20, 3:01 p.m.

Tick-tock, tick-tock, tick-tock . . . minutes rolled by, with the clock taunting us like a drill sergeant dishing out profanity. After much sitting, standing, pacing, and that annoying tingle of our legs falling asleep, we made it through. Finally, the important information we were waiting for came—though it came at the most peculiar of times. After a long wait, I had built up enough nerves, stress, and liquid intake that I was about ready to pee my pants. As the doctor told me the good news—that Harper succeeded in coming off ECMO—I got a pain in my bladder so sharp, I felt like I might pass out. I firmly told the neonatologist how happy I was with a look of pain on my face that could mean nothing good. All of this aside, Harper has come off of ECMO! Stability is on her side, and she seemingly had no complications during the procedure. However, she will remain open in her abdominal cavity with no plans of closing it surgically for possibly months to come. Donations are needed now more than ever. We have become so engrossed with CDH that we have been pushing to start our own nonprofit. The website will be up and running soon, and we will be helping other nonprofits take a firm grip on this disorder. As always, S4P and R4T!

Post 94:
September 20, 7:26 p.m.

Daddy again . . . All is quiet on the western front . . . and in Harper's room as well. The excitement has calmed and the nurses dispersed. Doctors, surgeons, respiratory therapists, and every other Tom, Dick, and Harry have vacated. All that remains in her room now are the idling obstacles of monitors, medications, and a ventilator, and, lastly, herself. As we sit here and watch her lay docile, the greenish-brown color of an un-ripened pumpkin, we wait, watch, and hope that her time remaining in the hospital will continue to show signs of improvement. S4P & R4T

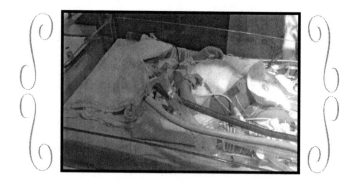

Post 95:
September 21, 12:48 p.m.

One hurdle down (ECMO), and several other hurdles spring up (dialysis and heparin). Thoughts of "When will it end?" fill our heads as we hear about one more machine and unfortunately the same blood thinner that helped her almost bleed out Wednesday of last week. Dialysis . . . of course the first thoughts that surface in any parent's mind are "For how long? Will this be a long-term thing? How will this affect her progression?" There are no real answers to this slew of questions, no pat on the back letting you know it will be okay—just the hard truth that your child has to trudge farther to the finish line. Doctors described to us the reasons why as we sat with heads in hands in disbelief. Due to her lack of kidney output, her lungs are struggling more with the amount of toxins in her system, thus there are signs of minimal regression in her lungs. Harper was put on the oscillator again for higher frequencies and pressures to hopefully open her lungs more. Heparin will be given to thin out the blood and help push the toxins to her kidneys more quickly. What do you say to a doctor as he tells you this? Nothing, no questions ever surface until they leave the room and then you wonder, "What did I just say okay to?" It is a feeling of overwhelming confusion due to the unsettling jargon that has just been blanketed over your mind. There is nothing more excruciatingly painful than watching a child in pain, until you see your child medically falling back. Regression . . . what a terrible term. I'm just glad Harper seems to be able to withstand anything. As always, S4P and R4T.

Post 96:
September 21, 4:05 p.m.

Massive machines, diligent doctors, and necessary nurses litter the room as we cast our eyes back and forth trying to make sense of all the chaos. There unfortunately is no set end date for the dialysis; however, the doctors are fairly certain there will not be any long-term effects. Harper continues to push through the pokes and prods with a calm but strong demeanor. Her mommy and I both attribute this to three things: the strength of all the love and prayers flooding her way, her stubbornness to not give in, and lastly, Hubert the giraffe, who stands by her side always through thick and thin, and his new friend, Hope the bunny, who keeps an eye on all that comes her way!

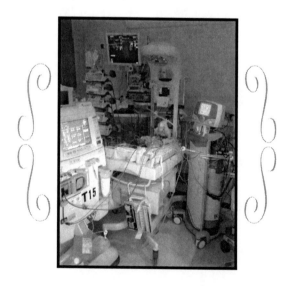

Post 97:
September 21, 8:21 p.m.

As the soft sounds of the oscillator churn away, Harper embraces the calming moments and attempts to regain some strength for tomorrow's hurdles. As for Mommy and me, we're plagued by raw nerves and heavy eyelids and are just fighting to stay upright. Thinking has become a luxury, as every minute keeps us on our toes. Knowing becomes hoping and hopes become prayers, as we have no idea what's in store for us or for Harper. They say that a war is never won because of one battle, nor one man; the war is won because the cause is unified for the greater good. Harper has a war that rages on, and you all—her friends and family—give us hope, because unified we are one. S4P & R4T

Post 98:
September 22, 1:21 p.m.

The human body is amazingly adaptive. It forces itself to mold and mend in response to situations that cause it harm. No one can deny that. However, when it alters its state too much because of a foreign body, it can start to harm itself. Harper's inability to release toxins, both foreign and domestic, is causing her body to combat itself. Jaundice, blood pressure issues, dialysis, lung regression, swelling—these are all terms that have plagued our minds today. Feeling as though you cannot do anything to better your child's situation is both terrifying and frustrating. Prayers, positive thoughts, and hope all help more than anyone could ever know, but the desire to wake up tomorrow and be told "Harper's ready to head home" is a constant ache. And it's a statement that I fear will be battles and heartaches away from this moment. At some point as a parent you have to ask yourself, "Who is really bettering whom?" R4T S4P

Post 99:
September 22, 3:34 p.m.

There is nothing more frightening than walking into your child's hospital room to discover her vitals plummeting. You enter the room with a blank stare, and the gazes of the people inside pierce you. The blood drains from your face as your heart races with tension, pain, and confusion. Doctors move from all corners of the room, grasping medications, "bagging" her, while others stand with their arms crossed, conversing about the next move. There is no calming feeling, no right or wrong answer, just acting. As we stood by her side, watching the stats flutter like wings and holding her to avoid further damage, all I could do was kiss her and assure her it would be okay. Minutes raced by as if time had stopped, and our hearts seemed to drop as she hit 48% of her normal 100% oxygen level . . . all we could do was watch. Sedation reigned over her body as we held her hands and prayed. Finally, 81 . . . 84 . . . 87 . . . 95 . . . 99 . . . 100. At last, Harper was soothed and comfortable, and everyone else present breathed a sigh of relief.

The drama had unfolded; the suspense had ceased. That is one stubborn-ass child, but God love her . . . S4P & R4T

Post 100:
September 22, 5:51 p.m.

As I sit here and listen to the shallow sounds of the oscillator and cast my eyes upon TooT, I find myself thinking of a little warrior who passed away yesterday. While I did not know him or his family personally, I did meet his father, Keith, and his big sister, Carolyn. What I gathered in our brief exchange of words was that Keith's son had fought for months, and in that period of time had helped to bring family, friends, and strangers together to share his journey. The mere mention of his name in the NICU brings nurses, doctors, and respiratory therapists to a smile and a tear. No words can soothe a parent whose child is in pain, nor make a parent feel at ease with the loss of a child. Tonight, barring anything major, we will not post anything about Harper; instead this will be Keith Barron Scott Jr.'s night. For what it's worth, I wish and hope that his smile rains upon Harper, and that his fight lives on in her. Goodnight, little guy.

Post 101:
September 23, 11:46 AM

Spirited . . . it sounds so much better than stubborn; however, it does not do Harper justice. TooT fights and exudes a degree of strength and resistance to sedatives that baffles physicians. Last night she had another fit like yesterday where her vitals plummeted. Doctors and nurses scrambled as they did before, however, this time they had sedation on hand. As her vitals went up and doctors convened, it was decided that she would have to be put on the maximum amount of sedation. Is it wrong that it made me feel a sense of hope that because she is such a fighter, she has to be sedated to the max? As the tension builds and the dialysis runs, surgeons are preparing themselves to change the dressings over her open wound— something Harper does not do well with. Even though she'll be sedated, the doctors are still uneasy about changing the gauze, for fear of agitating the fire-bellied baby. Thus they have decided to put her under a paralytic. Again, is it strange that I am proud of this? S4P & R4T

Post 102:
September 23, 4:59 p.m.

How does this happen? How can the patient determine what the doctor is doing by mere touch or the sound of his voice? Harper continues to battle day in and day out. I believe Harper would call this "suggestive medicine" if she knew the words. Consistently she tries to not only obstruct the airway of the oscillator by holding her breath, but also to combat the sedations with flailing arms. Minor surgery will be done tomorrow for a repair of the packing and dressings . . . if she will allow them . . . S4P & R4T

Post 103:
September 24, 12:34 a.m.

As the minutes tick away and Hubert and Hope calmly watch on, Harper rests for her surgery in the a.m. The night has been filled with vital ups and downs and the clip-clap of the nurses running around to address the issues at hand. While there is no direct correlation between her "episodes," there is a consensus among the nurses that brings a bit of sadness: she is in pain. Bolus after bolus, tantrum after episode, they stand and watch, determine and convene, but ultimately her comfort is their utmost concern. Tomorrow will be another long day for TooT . . . much like the days prior. Just a bit longer . . . I promise . . . just a little bit . . . S4P & R4T

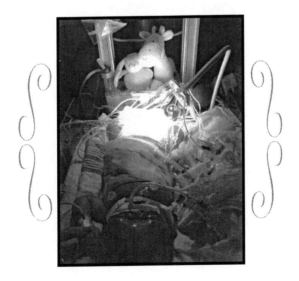

Post 104:
September 24, 11:57 a.m.

White noise . . . the sounds of the room become all too familiar and too easy to drown out. The sight of the lurking machines numbs your emotions, bogging them down, making you unable to cry. Doctors see your eyes and ask if everything is okay. Of course you nod and affirm that nothing is wrong, but everyone in the room knows you're full of it. Voices bounce off of each other like bumper cars and again you are told, "We will have her back to you shortly." "Shortly" becomes an aching eternity and there is no sense of relief. Your daughter lies there, open for all to see, vulnerable. She is bleeding lightly, as if her body is crying red tears. As a parent all you can say is, "Be strong, baby, they just need to change your dressings and clean you up." S4P & R4T

Post 105:
September 24, 4:30 p.m.

Lines . . . not the kind you stare at as they jive up and down, communicating vital signs, but rather the waiting kind, the kind filled with machines, doctors, and nurses all waiting to perform tests on a bed of innocence. We cut our way to the front of the line to see Harper. Test after test, we watch on, seeing the vitals fluctuate, patiently burning a hole through the monitors with our eyes as we await their verdicts. She holds my index finger in her small hand, grasping it with a force only a survivor could muster. Soft words, breaths, and smiles rain down upon her as Mommy and I try to ease her pain. As her vitals rise to a positive state, we are pulled aside for an explanation of what is in store for Harper tomorrow. Dialysis of course is becoming a word used all too frequently, transfusion . . . not so much. Descriptions of different toxins surface in the conversation as we are told that a major transfusion is in store . . . S4P & R4T

Post 106:
September 24, 7:19 p.m.

Harper has been silently sleeping and continues to do so. While we have some time, here are some questions people have asked, and we thought we would answer. :)

Q: Do you have any idea the impact your family has made on the world? You guys are amazing. Every day, to see the faith, the love, the hope, and you share it with us! Do you know how amazing that makes you; it means you truly let God's light shine through! And moreover, the fact that you post things wanting to know about our lives. Do you know how great that is?

A: Honestly, we have no idea what degree of "impact" we have had. The main goal we set when starting this page was to allow our friends and family to be "up to speed" on what was going on with Harper. However, when people started frequenting the page, we began to make it a point to help raise awareness in any way we could. We have been maintaining the page as a way to interact with you all and to bring prayers and positive thoughts to our little girl, because every little bit helps. In terms of why we want to know about you all, it is because without you and your constant help, we would not have the strength to keep going. You all are unbelievably important to us and to Harper's progression. We love you all.

Q: Was Harper diagnosed in the womb or after she was born? Do they attribute her condition to simply genetics or other possible causes?

A: Harper was diagnosed in the womb. She was diagnosed on April, 25 (at 24 weeks) after the ultrasound. Our OBGYN at the time took us into our room and insisted we see a perinatal specialist, and at the time we thought it was something small and could be easily fixed . . . Unfortunately, we were wrong. In terms of attributing the disorder to genetics or any other direct causes, there is not enough evidence in the research being done to pinpoint it to one thing or the other (which is something we eventually want to change!).

Q: Are there any specific needs or challenges that you face as a family that we can help you with? We are ALL here to support you and your sweet family in any way that we possibly can! Although some may not be able to donate at this time, I'm sure they'd love to offer any kind of assistance they can to help you get through your tough time. Sending love and hope.

A: First off, we thank each and every one of you for your contributions. Prayers, positive thoughts, donations, heartfelt gifts—they all have helped immensely. In terms of something more to contribute, we want to leave that up to you. As we are new parents, we have no idea what we will need down the road. As for something specific—spread awareness! Tell a friend or family member or share it on your page. You all have been doing an unbelievable job at that.

Q: What did you do when she was first diagnosed? Feelings, treatment, everything. I couldn't be as strong as you both are.
A: What did we do when she was first diagnosed? Honestly, we just did what the OB/GYN said: got an appointment with the perinatal specialist. At the time, we had no idea what all of this was going to amount to, and the way we were approached about it by our OB/GYN was that it was nothing detrimental. Of course this all happened right after the ultrasound, so we were mostly thrilled to see our Little TooT. We were basically enveloped in sense of joy tempered by minor caution.

Q: What is one thing that you wish for Harper given how sick she has been?

A: Obviously, we want her to get better and not have

any long-lasting effects. Beyond that, I, Daddy, wish more than anything that she will one day be able to run a marathon and defy all kinds of odds to do things they say a child with CDH could never do. As for Mommy, she wants her to be a boxer, because she always has arms flailing and can handle a large amount of pain. Most of all, we both hope that she will live a long, fulfilling life, and may one day become an advocate for CDH and help spread the word!

Post 107:
September 25, 11:53 a.m.

Transfusion—it is essentially replacing the old, toxin-infested blood with clean, oxygenated blood, giving a euphoric feeling to most patients. Euphoria . . . it sounds almost too good to be true for TooT. We hope as parents that our children never endure intense pain, nor know the misery of heartache, even though these are the forces that develop children into stronger and more driven human beings. Of course, that same strength enables children to drive their parents crazy later on in life, something I cannot wait to endure. Harper, you deserve every sense of happiness that a transfusion can produce . . . S4P & R4T

Post 108:
September 25, 4:59 p.m.

Nephrologists, neonatologists, pediatric surgeons,

NICU nurses—the list goes on. It was a barrage of multiple consonants and vowels discussing the clotted line within her neck. Of course the question, "Do you have any questions?" shortly followed, and as usual, the overwhelming vocabulary and stares made us draw a blank. After digesting copious amounts of information, we can tell you this: the line that parades all of the medications for dialysis and the transfusion into her body is most likely clogged. Thus we'll almost certainly have to draw another line through her groin. While it is necessary, it is both aggravating and unsettling to hear. I guess my protective nature is surfacing, and I selfishly want to hold TooT . . . S4P & R4T

Post 109:
September 25, 10:20 p.m.

People say that children have the universal language. Crying, whining, smiling, pouting—they all amount to some form of body language. Adults combine a slew of words, whether in ecstasy or bitter anger, to amplify and enhance the emotions surfacing from within. So what do you say to an infant who cannot verbalize her emotions, let alone her pain? You regurgitate the normal "Calm down, it's okay," even though you know you could say anything, and just the sound of your voice is all she needs. As a first-time father, I am discovering the key element is touch. Harper continues to try to combat the oscillator by attempting to breathe over the machine, causing respiratory distress and lowering her vitals. Arms flail and face gestures change as TooT's mommy and I hold her hands and calm her down, only to find out the best thing about this is that she did not need her sedation to get her over the hump. ;) S4P & R4T

Post 110:
September 26, 12:19 p.m.

Time is an element that unfortunately escapes us in the blink of an eye. From the sandy-eyed mornings to the blanket-diving nights, the majority of people go about their day toward a common goal of giving themselves the best chance of succeeding. Difficulties spring up daily, and labors yield achievements, but most people never stop and take a look at the simple gifts around them. The time we have with others is seemingly taken for granted; not many look at the ability to breathe or walk as a privilege. I am not a martyr by any sense, but as Harper wiggles and throws her hands about (as if to lead a riot), I cannot help but be reminded that every second I have with her is a blessing. Days are too long, and hours don't compare; the seconds count. As the noise of the dialysis machine carries throughout the confines of her room and the sedation monitor's lights (of which there are fewer now, by the way!) blink, casting awkward shadows on the walls, I smile and remain thankful for every wiggle, every second, of every day . . . S4P & R4T

Post 111:
September 26, 7:15 p.m.

Everyone has that moment that changes his or her life. For some, it's their first "big-person job," for others, their first house, or the day their child was born. I too perceive these as monumental events; however, nothing equates to the emotional high I received from holding Harper for the first time ever today. My walk into the room seemed just as long and obstacle ridden as ever, and, per usual, people littered the room. They smiled at us like children waiting to yell "Surprise!" at a birthday party. Only the words we would hear would far exceed any birthday tidings: "Today you both get to hold Miss Harper!" Our faces lit up like the Fourth of July, followed by questions of "Really?" and "Are you serious?" Upon getting the shock out of our systems, we prepared for the most incredible experience of our lives. Minutes were not enough, and the hour seemed to melt away as we coddled, cuddled, and kissed our angel, our everything, our TooT . . . :)
S4P & R4T

Post 112:
September 27, 11:47 a.m.

Before Harper, the phrase "defying the odds" called to my mind pictures of famous sports moments. For most, that won't be surprising, as I am male. Despite the obvious differences, Harper and those athletes have a pivotal similarity: will. Will drives a person to overcome odds and discrimination, to face the last few, seemingly impossible seconds. In Harper's case, she is fighting for the will to live. Many athletes never have to fight that battle, and never know that kind of will. Yesterday, we held our daughter for the first time. Today, she shows added resilience and even more fight. Love for family far outweighs the will to win, but they do go hand in hand to an extent, wouldn't you agree? Today Miss TooT's oxygen levels are down to 50% assistance! Not to mention her sedation levels are lowering and she had no tantrums last night, which meant no boluses (sedation)! Her wiggles have caused hardly any saturation on her dressings, which means she is healing better! The only thing to hold our breaths for today is that her central line (where her medications and nutrients go) will be moved to her femoral artery in her groin. However, we all know she's got this in the bag! R4T & S4P

Post 113:
September 27, 6:22 p.m.

Mommy and I walked into the room to find a wiggling, squirming, partially sedated yet active little bundle— otherwise known as Harper. Scrub-clad bodies, gloved hands, and an array of medical tools obstructed our path through her room, and the beeping of light-covered boxes and discussions of the femoral central line blended into a constant mutter. To nobody's surprise, Harper could care less about anything going on. TooT tossed and wriggled without tears, exuding a cuteness that put her mother and me at ease and left smiles on our faces. Medically speaking, today was a good day. Since yesterday, Harper has been showing signs of progress, and while they are baby steps (no pun intended), they are pushes in the right direction. Harper now has a femoral central line for medication and a dialysis line in her neck. She has steadily performed at 50-55% oxygen assistance and continues to put out small amounts of urine (PRAY FOR PEE, by the way!). Her sedation levels are still being reduced, and she was a very good girl during her procedure today! :) S4P & R4T

Post 114:
September 28, 12:49 p.m.

Our tenacious TooT is at it again! Through the struggles, trials, and tribulations, one would think that something or someone so petite would cave. Adults cringe at the thought of pain, and unfortunately are sometimes the source of it. Harper teaches us daily, not how to read, write, color or count, but how to wake up a better person. To smile, to cry, to be saddened or hopeful—these are the marks that only love can leave. TooT has brought love and amiability into the households and hearts of so many, and for this I do not know if I could ever repay her . . . Today TooT has again needed less oxygen assistance! We are down to 30%! Dialysis is at it again and will be for many days to come, but she is tolerating it very well today. She was a good TooT overnight and did not need any extra sedation; in fact, she is being weaned down from taking methadone (a strong sedative) every 4 hours to every 6! She's also needing less and less nitric gas to help with her blood flow! She peed 4 ml of fluid overnight, which was better than all of yesterday combined (the praying for pee seems to be working). However, the biggest step of all . . . she is calming herself down without sedatives when she gets agitated and uncomfortable! S4P & R4T

Post 115:
September 28, 6:59 p.m.

Drops of rain litter the air and the sky is painted grey; a storm moves in, and sleepiness accompanies. Mommy and I are steadfast on our Google binge, watching the time melt away as Harper lies peacefully sleeping. Her hands awkwardly open for no particular reason, as if she's dreaming about unintentionally grabbing and breaking the items Mommy and I cherish most. A sense of serenity fills the room as we pass the time, not in a state of worry, but in a state of simply being—being here for our most precious gift, Harper. Another big moment for Harper today: she finally got to ingest some breast milk! While it was through a drip line, it was a huge step. Hopefully her bowel reacts well, because there is the potential for infection (her bowel has not had to be very active, which means the bacteria in her intestine will need to react well for it to not stress). We have also been able to give it to her orally via Q-tip, so she can taste it. Vent settings are steadily lower than they were yesterday . . . Remember, everything has to be done in baby steps. :) Otherwise, today has been a very easygoing and somewhat rainy day. :)

Post 116:
September 29, 1:51 p.m.

Smack, smack, smack . . . Little TooT is fast at work licking the Q-tip as we introduce her to the taste of Mommy's milk. Dialysis will as usual be filling several hours of TooT's day, but I know she will be able to nonchalantly get through it! As she champions through another medicine–imbued day, we are told that again she will be weaned. Today they will be reducing her mean pressure (the pressure exerted by a machine to keep her lungs open and operating). It's a small reduction, from 24 to 23, but remember, baby steps! Because she has showed such stability, Mommy and I will be having a little day out and about. We promise to update you tonight after we come spend a bit more time with Miss TooT! We love you all and hope you understand! Remember, R4T & S4P.

Post 117:
September 30, 12:22 a.m.

After a much-needed day of seemingly carefree ease and relaxation, Mommy and I strolled back into the room of our beautiful Little TooT. With a new owl sticker upon her right cheek and a wiggle that screamed "adorable," Harper was excited to hear our voices. News of progress filled our ears. We were told that she is down to 25% now on her oxygen assistance. Dopamine is being steadily reduced every hour, and she is continuing to calm herself down without a bolus. While the hour is late and darkness blankets the room, TooT still finds a way to show us that in the end, she will be okay. S4P & R4T

Post 118:
September 30, 4:41 p.m.

After a morning of positives, the afternoon inspires less enthusiasm. Doctors cannot pinpoint why Harper's kidneys are failing. Iron was the apparent cause of this failure, or so they thought. Long-term dialysis is looking more and more likely, as TooT is struggling to pee. Three milliliters yesterday were lowered to 1 ml today, as the medication has ceased to work. With that battle heightening, other positives have become more apparent. Harper could be off of dopamine (helps with blood pressure); however, doctors want to maintain small levels to help her kidneys. Harper's nitric levels have dropped as well from 10 to 5. Mean pressures continue to lower at small increments, but remember, baby steps. Please pray for our TooT! Her kidneys need to kick it into high gear! S4P & R4T

Post 119:
September 30, 10:23 p.m.

Tonight . . . As Harper lay unsettled and fighting the oscillator, we conversed with a doctor about our miracle that is TooT. Feelings of joy shakily balanced on a fence between hope and despair as we discussed what we do know and what could be. Lacking answers, the questions darted left and right. We still do not know the reasons why her kidneys are failing. Theories seem to be as unsettling as "I don't know," and for the first time I felt not anger but disappointment. Harper fights tooth and nail, and I feel as though we should be able to do more. I guess I feel a sense of disappointment in myself . . . Otherwise, she continues her weaning down from dopamine and her vent settings . . .
Pray. Please.

Post 120:
October 1, 1:16 p.m.

Today while there were no major changes, there was a new concern: a high white blood cell count, or possible infection. They do not know the root of the infection or the severity of it. While this is another obstacle, I saw the infection as an analogy. As weird as it seems, it makes me think of TooT as a beautiful, little, infectious nugget that has invaded all of our hearts. I know she will overcome the trials that lie ahead . . .
S4P & R4T

Post 121:

October 1, 9:17 p.m.

After work, the plan was for me to go down to the hospital after I had changed and gotten a bite of food. But instead, I got off early: "You're cut!" No words could have been sweeter to my ears. All I could think about at work (besides the fact that I hadn't eaten in a while) was Harper. Every time I looked at the clock, it seemed to have turned back 30 minutes. As I raced to leave, I got a call from Erin before I could get out the door: "Are you off? Because they are going to let us hold her again!" After my heart started beating again, it was going a mile a minute. Traffic was horrific, as it always is in times of anticipation. But parking wasn't so bad. I raced upstairs, washed up, entered the NICU, got stopped by family for a quick "Hey," and this is what I walked into.

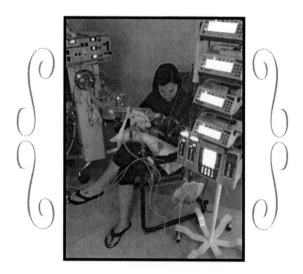

By the way, Harper is doing okay. They hope to pinpoint her possible infection, and that could take a few days. But she is staying at low settings on her vent and she is snug in Mommy's arms. :)

Post 122:
October 1, 9:50 p.m.

Melts my heart to see Daddy lovin' on our sweet Little TooT. :)

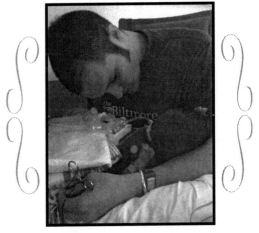

Post 123:
October 2, 11:42 a.m.

Mom reporting today while Dad is at work this morning. Feeling truly blessed to be surprised yet again with the news that we get to hold TooT. My feet have yet to come back to earth after the wonderful feeling of having her in my arms.
There is not much to relay this morning. She is having her dialysis as usual right now. She had a bit of an episode earlier and required a bolus of sedation, but

other than that, not much has changed with the little one. There have been talks of putting on a wound vac to replace the current dressing. This will help pull the skin together and promote the growth of new skin cells over top of the material inside of her (which will disintegrate eventually). It will also limit the number of times the dressing will need to get changed, which makes for a happy TooT.

As always, S4P & R4T.

Post 124:
October 2, 8:41 p.m.

Confirmation . . . there is nothing more adorable than seeing your child cuddled up looking like a burrito. As TooT snuggles up, Mommy and I quietly discuss pictures of years past with a few family members. As a parent, I can safely say, I hope I never have to go through the things with Harper that I made my parents suffer through as a child. Ken dolls and a lighted grill don't mix. Tonight, Harper had her catheter removed. There was, unfortunately, no point to having it in, as she has still not peed. The oxygen assistance remains at around 30%. However, her blood gases have not been up to par, so her pressures needed to be increased on her oscillator. Her liver is producing massive amounts of bilirubin (which is the pigment found in bile and makes her skin yellowish) and is having difficulty functioning. Hang in there, Little TooT . . . S4P & R4T

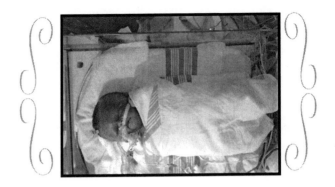

Post 125:
October 3, 2:22 p.m.

Crying . . . this is all I can post . . . my notes. I'm sorry.

Lungs:
One to keep expanded, she is on 24
50 down to 32 on her delta
20 down to 4 on nitric
CDH has impeded the left lung growth.
Kidneys:
Always struggled
Lasiks were given at the max levels.
Hemofiltration on ECMO.
Potassium levels are essential for normal cell growth
in the kidneys and for excretions.
Dialysis is not working.
Kidneys are in failure.
Why is she failing?
What are the chances they will come back and make
urine?
What do you think has caused this issue?
Iron issues?

Liver:

Iron L: 200 could cause liver toxicity.

Not being fed can cause issues.

TPN can cause issues in the liver enzymes.

Hypoxic: less oxygen in the body.

Ongoing question, should we continue?

Transferrin is high, which binds the iron.

Ferritin levels at 53,198. The normal is 150.

Increase in stress, iron, infections, big concern.

Bilirubin, cholestasis . . . iron, lack of feed, feed needs to increase, phenobarbital, ECMO for three plus weeks. Where are we going?

Kidneys are the most life-threatening thing. IRON!

Ventilation is a huge concern, lung growth, only time can do that.

Lung issues, ECMO timeframe seems to be a root cause. She has less than 50% chance of survival and possibly much less. No transplant can be discussed while all of this is going on. If things do not get better in the short term, we have our answer: she will not make it.

Post 126:
October 4, 1:44 p.m.

As Michelle, Harper's respiratory therapist, said, "People do not realize how much of a miracle a healthy child is. The fact that all of those cells reproduce and align so well is truly a miracle." It is hard to grasp that fact when your child remains in a healthy state. Even in Harper's state, it is difficult for Mommy and me to realize. We see nothing but perfection in our Little TooT. We have had a different experience than many parents, and it has made us realize how true Michelle's statement really is. We ask for all of you parents to take a step back and do something loving for your child today. If it is nothing more than telling your child you love them, realize that they are not just any miracle, they are your miracle. Harper's blood pressure is unstable at the max amount of dopamine, so epinephrine had to be added before dialysis. As far as vent settings, liver issues, and kidney prognosis, they remain as they were yesterday.

TooT, our little angel . . .

S4P & R4T

Post 127:
October 4, 8:16 p.m.

Miss Harper is becoming a baby fashionista. :) Personally, this is my favorite of the bows (Daddy) . . . This and the fish one.

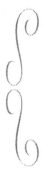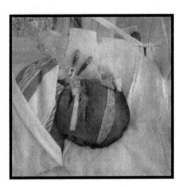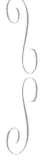

She is staying stable on her settings; however, they have had to administer epinephrine again for blood pressure :(

Post 128:
October 5, 1:56 p.m.

Difficult times for Harper thus far today . . . Her heart rate dropped into the 60s for 6 minutes today, and the doctors don't know exactly why. They were able to manage blood clots in her catheter, and due to the heart rate drop, they increased her epinephrine drip. When this all happened, dialysis had to stop. An echo of her heart was performed and it showed no clots in her heart . . . thank God. As expected, her blood pressure dropped as well during this time, but recovered. Her pH was low, so the ventilator settings had to go up. Her chest X-ray didn't show signs of change. As far as the kidneys and liver go, they remain plagued by iron and still are in a state of acute failure. S4P & R4T
We need you now, Big Guy . . . everyone please pray.

Post 129:
October 5, 7:46 p.m.

Due to issues with her last remaining catheter entry being clogged, dialysis could not be performed today. It was the closest call we have had since the fourth surgery. Without dialysis entry, the toxicity of iron and fluid in her body will not be manageable. We are told that the surgeons are not sure how much longer the catheter in her neck will last. This is me reading Harper the book "The Stinky Cheese Man and other Fairly Stupid Tales" as we patiently waited for news on whether the catheter could still be used or not. Please pray hard these next few days, as they are some of the most telling days for our beautiful angel, TooT.

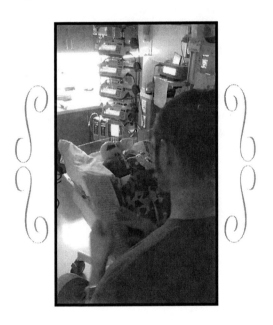

Post 130:
October 6, 1:46 p.m.

A father has to be a provider, a teacher, a role model, but most importantly, a distant authority figure who can never be pleased. Otherwise, how will children ever understand the concept of God?
— Stephen Colbert

But seriously . . .

As a father, I have learned more since August 20th than I have learned in a quarter of a century. Not in the normal sense of learning . . . I guess you could call it "adaptive changing." Harper made me adapt and change to become a better man, person, and most of all father. Without her, I would never know unconditional love and the stresses that it brings. Today she will undergo her last shot. Dialysis is the most important treatment right now, as the toxicity has to be taken out of her system in order for her to survive. A 24-hour continuous dialysis has been implemented instead of the 3-4 hour sittings daily. That being said, it will put more stress on the catheter in her neck, which is barely usable as is. Our nephrologist has told us that if this does not work, we are out of options.

We need a miracle.

S4P & R4T

Post 131:
October 6, 6:59 p.m.

We are back on dialysis; however, we will all be holding our breath for a while, as she will have to be on it for days. The catheter that the dialysis is using is the last line of defense for Harper. If the catheter clots, we have no other entry line. The 24-hour dialysis is more susceptible to clots in the catheter lines, but it has to be done. Pray, kneel, bow, do whatever you all have been doing! It has all worked thus far!

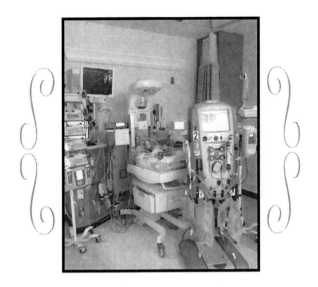

Post 132:
October 6, 10:22 p.m.

We love you all . . .

Post 133:
October 7, 4:18 AM

Tonight heaven gained a beautiful angel. I love you, Harper. You taught me what love is. Goodnight, sweet pea. Daddy and Mommy love you . . .

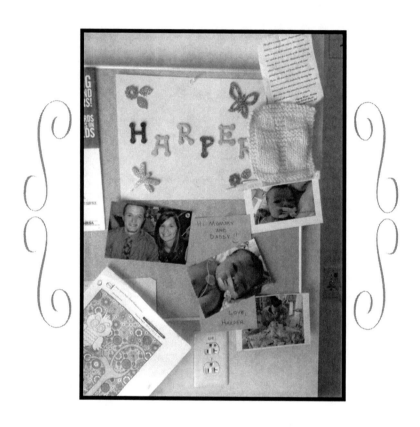

Saying Goodbye

Harper passed away in our arms. Wrapped in a blanket, snuggled between Mommy and me, she slipped away quickly, in just under a minute and a half.

As we both kissed Harper's forehead and each other, we cried not out of pain, misery, or anger, but out of an unsettling joy. She would no longer feel the sensation of a tube puffing her lungs up and down, or of an open wound, or of struggle of any kind. She was going home. I say "home" not in the sense of four walls, a ceiling, and floor, but to be with her family and friends in a heavenly place, wherever that may be.

As I type and cry and feel a sense of sorrow, I pray she will always be with me. Mommy and Daddy love you, baby, always and forever. You will always be our first, our child, our everything.

A Note from the Editors about CDH

A congenital diaphragmatic hernia (CDH) is a life-threatening birth defect in which the diaphragm fails to form fully, resulting in a hole through which abdominal organs can pass into the chest cavity and obstruct the lungs. It occurs in one out of every 2,500 births. In the United States, roughly 1,600 babies are born each year with CDH, and globally, there is a child born every ten minutes with this condition. Of these, only about 50 percent survive, and many of those who do survive suffer difficult medical complications.

Although CDH is nearly as common as spina bifida and cystic fibrosis, it remains a relatively unknown condition, and as a result, receives little funding and research. Some parents of children affected by CDH are working to raise awareness of this condition. It was to this end that *Harper* was compiled and published. If you are moved by what you have read, please help spread the word about this debilitating and deadly birth defect by sharing and recommending this book, talking to friends and health professionals, and donating to a CDH fund-raising organization if you can.

There are several U.S. nonprofits dedicated to raising awareness and funding for CDH family support and medical research, and any donation is a step forward on the path to better and more reliable treatments. With enough contributions, perhaps one day, children like Harper will have a greater than fifty-fifty chance of survival.

A few CDH awareness organizations:

Cherubs
Association of CDH Research, Awareness
    and Support
3650 Rogers Road #290
Wake Forest, NC 27587
www.cherubs-cdh.org

Breath of Hope, Inc.
Virginia
www.breathofhopeinc.com

Global CDH
P.O. Box 175
Hasbrouck Heights, NJ 07604
www.globalcdh.org

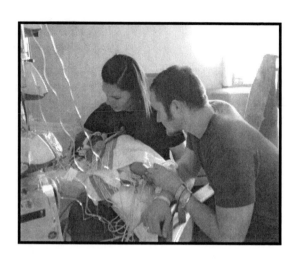

About the Author

Upon graduating from the University of Virginia, William Stanfield returned to work in the restaurant industry. A few years prior to the writing of this book, he met Erin Byers, Harper's mother and the love of his life. They remain together today, very much in love, and will always love and remember their firstborn daughter, Harper Ann Stanfield. This is William's first book.

CPSIA information can be obtained at www.ICGtesting.com
Printed in the USA
LVOW07s1626110514

385318LV00001B/169/P